Be.Bull

Workout

Book

for

Men

Be.Bull

Workout Book for Men

450 Workouts
to
Lose Fat and Build Muscle

Be.Bull Publishing Group

Toronto, Canada

Authors:

Be.Bull Publishing Group

Mauricio Vasquez & Devon Abbruzzese

First Printing: December 2021

ISBN- 978-1-990709-64-7

FREE DOWNLOAD

BONUS No 1

ALL LOGGING SHEETS from this book are available *FOR NO EXTRA COST* for you by scanning a QR code.

You can scan the QR code, print, and record your workouts to measure your performance as many times as you want.

(The QR is found on the following pages)

BONUS No 2 -

VIDEOS for ALL EXERCISES ARE AVAILABLE to check how the exercises are to be performed

(The QR codes are found at the end of this book)

Unlock Your Fitness Potential
with Artificial Intelligence

I am thrilled to introduce a groundbreaking tool, *"AI-Powered Training Coach" GPT*, for physical fitness, developed with the latest advancements in AI technology. This advanced tool is designed to enhance your workout experience, offering personalized exercise plans tailored to your preferences, needs, and the equipment you have available.

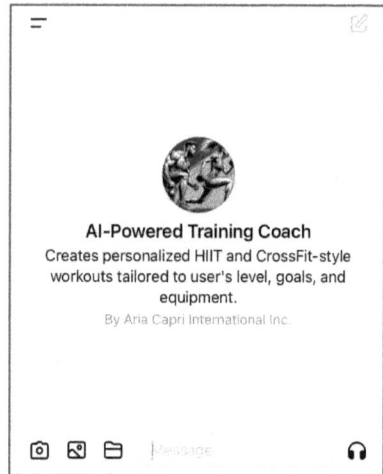

AI-Powered Training Coach
Creates personalized HIIT and CrossFit-style workouts tailored to user's level, goals, and equipment.
By Aria Capri International Inc.

This innovative AI system, utilizing Generative Pre-trained Transformer (GPT) technology by OpenAI.com, is specifically programmed to support your fitness journey. It acts as a dynamic fitness companion, aligning with your personal fitness goals and the resources at your disposal, providing custom-tailored workout routines and fitness advice.

Engaging with this AI tool is incredibly user-friendly and intuitive. Upon access, you'll be presented with a straightforward interface where you can input your fitness objectives, available equipment, and other relevant details. The AI processes this information rapidly, delivering tailored workout plans and suggestions almost instantly.

Whether your goal is to build muscle, increase endurance, or simply maintain a healthy lifestyle, this AI tool is your gateway to a more effective and personalized fitness experience.

Included in this section there are a couple of screenshots displaying the user interface you'll encounter when accessing this unique fitness AI tool. This visual guide offers a clear overview of the tool's functionality, assisting you in your first steps towards a smarter, AI-enhanced workout regimen.

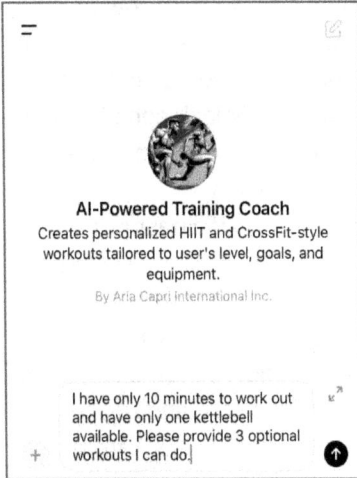

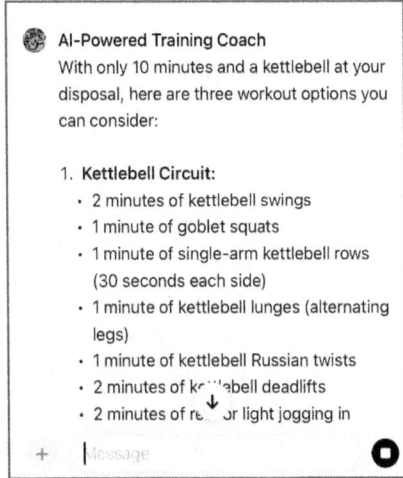

AI-Powered Training Coach
Creates personalized HIIT and CrossFit-style workouts tailored to user's level, goals, and equipment.
By Aria Capri International Inc.

I have only 10 minutes to work out and have only one kettlebell available. Please provide 3 optional workouts I can do.

AI-Powered Training Coach
With only 10 minutes and a kettlebell at your disposal, here are three workout options you can consider:

1. **Kettlebell Circuit:**
   - 2 minutes of kettlebell swings
   - 1 minute of goblet squats
   - 1 minute of single-arm kettlebell rows (30 seconds each side)
   - 1 minute of kettlebell lunges (alternating legs)
   - 1 minute of kettlebell Russian twists
   - 2 minutes of kettlebell deadlifts
   - 2 minutes of rest or light jogging in

To embark on your journey towards achieving your fitness goals with the support of this innovative AI technology, please go to this link
https://mindscapeartwork.ck.page/trainingcoachgpt
or scan this QR code.

Disclaimer

1. Be.Bull Publishing (Aria Capri International Inc.) strongly recommends that you consult with your physician before beginning any exercise program or workout. You should be in good physical condition and be able to participate in the exercises and workouts. We are not a licensed medical care provider and represents that we have no expertise in diagnosing, examining, or treating medical conditions of any kind, or in determining the effect of any specific exercise or workout on a medical condition.

2. You should understand that when participating in any exercise or workout, there is the possibility of physical injury. If you engage in the exercises and workouts of this book, you agree that you do so at your own risk, are voluntarily participating in these activities, assume all risk of injury to yourself, and agree to release and discharge Be.Bull Publishing (Aria Capri International Inc.) from any and all claims or causes of action, known or unknown, arising out of this book and videos.

3. The information provided is not intended to be a substitute for professional medical advice, diagnosis or treatment. Never disregard professional medical advice, or delay in seeking it, because of something you have read on this book or watch in the videos. Never rely on information on this book or videos in place of seeking professional medical advice.

4. Be.Bull Publishing (Aria Capri International Inc.) is not responsible or liable for any advice, course of treatment, diagnosis or any other information, services or products that you obtain through this book or videos. You are encouraged to consult with your doctor with regard to the information contained on or through this book or videos. After reading this book or watching videos from this book, you are encouraged to review the information carefully with your professional healthcare provider.

Go to the link or scan the QR code shown below to check out other workout books

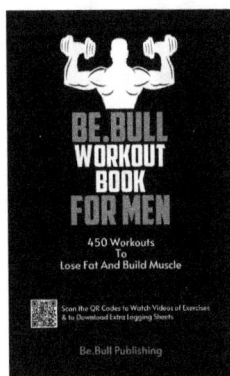

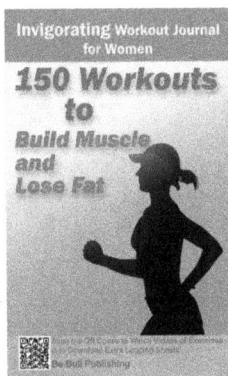

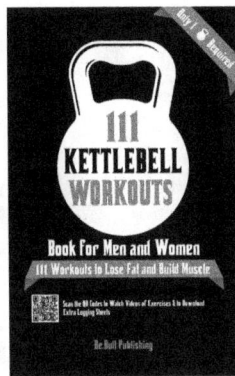

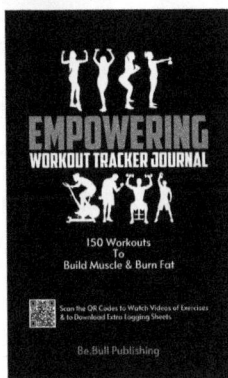

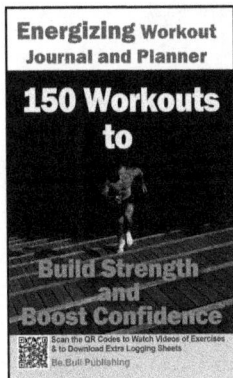

BE.BULL WORKOUT BOOK FOR MEN
450 Workouts To Lose Fat And Build Muscle
Scan the QR Codes to Watch Videos of Exercises & to Download Extra Logging Sheets
Be.Bull Publishing

Invigorating Workout Journal for Women
150 Workouts to Build Muscle and Lose Fat
Be.Bull Publishing

111 KETTLEBELL WORKOUTS
Book For Men and Women
111 Workouts to Lose Fat and Build Muscle
Scan the QR Codes to Watch Videos of Exercises & to Download Extra Logging Sheets
Be.Bull Publishing

EMPOWERING WORKOUT TRACKER JOURNAL
150 Workouts To Build Muscle & Burn Fat
Scan the QR Codes to Watch Videos of Exercises & to Download Extra Logging Sheets
Be.Bull Publishing

Energizing Workout Journal and Planner
150 Workouts to Build Strength and Boost Confidence
Scan the QR Codes to Watch Videos of Exercises & to Download Extra Logging Sheets
Be.Bull Publishing

https://linktr.ee/be.bull

BONUS No 1 - **ALL LOGGING SHEETS of this book are available through this QR code** that you can use to **scan, print, and record your workouts to measure your performance** as many times you want

Work-outs	Day 1 Reps / Time / Weight	Day 2 Reps / Time / Weight	Day 3 Reps / Time / Weight	Day 4 Reps / Time / Weight	Day 5 Reps / Time / Weight
1 Complete as many rounds as possible in 12 minutes of: - 3 rope climbs - 12 push presses - 50 single-unders					
2 Complete as many rounds as possible in 12 minutes of: - 6 squat cleans - 6 pull-ups					
3 7 Rounds for time: - 400 meter run - 20 walking lunges - 15 pull-ups - 5 burpees					
4 5 Rounds for time of: - 500-meter run - 20 overhead squats					
5 As many reps as possible in 30 minutes: - 5 deadlifts - 15 push-ups - 10 box jumps					
6 As many reps as possible in 20 minutes: - 7 dumbbell man makers - 8 box step ups					
7 As many reps as possible in 15 minutes: - 30 double-unders - 15 power snatches					

	Day 1	Day 2	Day 3	Day 4	Day 5
Work-outs	Reps / Time / Weight	Reps / Time / Weight	Reps / Time / Weight	Reps / Time / Weight	Reps / Time / Weight
8 Every minute on the minute for 20 minutes: - 5 thrusters - 5 burpees					
9 For time: - 100 curtis p's one "curtis p" complex is comprised of one power clean, one lunge (each leg), and one push press.					
10 As many reps as possible in 15 minutes: - 5 pendlay rows - 10 strict curls - 15 push-ups					
11 Complete as many rounds as possible in 21 minutes of: - 21 bench presses - 21 assisted pull-ups - 21 sit-ups					
12 For time: 10,9,8... 3,2,1 of - chest-to-Bar Pull-Ups - box jumps - straight leg sit-ups					
13 5 Rounds for time: - 15 air squats - 15 burpees - 15 hand release push-ups					

Work-outs	Day 1 Reps / Time / Weight	Day 2 Reps / Time / Weight	Day 3 Reps / Time / Weight	Day 4 Reps / Time / Weight	Day 5 Reps / Time / Weight
14 As many reps as possible in 20 minutes: - 30 box jumps - 20 push presses - 30 pull-ups					
15 For time: 21-15-9 - kettlebell swings - rows					
16 With a pair of dumbbells, 4 rounds for time of: - 25-meter weighted lunge - 175-meter farmers carry					
17 21-18-15-12-9-6-3 Reps for time: - thrusters - bar facing burpees					
18 As many reps as possible in 27 minutes: from 0:00-10:00: 1 mile run - max clean-and-jerks rest from 10:00-13:00 from 13:00-20:00: - 800 meter run - max power snatches rest from 20:00-23:00 from 23:00-27:00: - 400 meter run - max thrusters					

	Day 1	Day 2	Day 3	Day 4	Day 5
Work-outs	Reps / Time / Weight	Reps / Time / Weight	Reps / Time / Weight	Reps / Time / Weight	Reps / Time / Weight
19 6 Rounds for time: - 9 thrusters - 9 pull-ups					
20 In 10 minutes, complete as much as possible of: - 1 deadlift - 50-m run - 2 deadlifts - 100-m run - 3 deadlifts - 150-m run - 4 deadlifts - 200-m run etc.					
21 On a 25-minute clock, 5 rounds of: - row for 50 seconds, rest 10 seconds - row for 40 seconds, rest 20 seconds - row for 30 seconds, rest 30 seconds - row for 20 seconds, rest 40 seconds - row for 10 seconds, rest 50 seconds					

	Day 1	Day 2	Day 3	Day 4	Day 5
Work-outs	**Reps / Time / Weight**	**Reps / Time / Weight**	**Reps / Time / Weight**	**Reps / Time / Weight**	**Reps / Time / Weight**
22 For time: - 40 kettlebell snatches - 20 calorie ski - 40 kettlebell goblet squats - 20 calorie ski - 40 kettlebell clean-and-presses - 20 calorie ski - 40 kettlebell swings - 20 calorie ski					
23 For time: - 30 devil presses - 60 dumbbell thrusters - 90 burpees					
24 For time: - 30 walking lunge steps - 30 assisted pull-ups - 30 box jumps - 30 single-unders - 30 back extensions - 30 assisted push-ups - 30 hanging knee raises - 30 wall-ball - 30 sit-ups - 10 rope climbs					

Work-outs	Day 1 Reps / Time / Weight	Day 2 Reps / Time / Weight	Day 3 Reps / Time / Weight	Day 4 Reps / Time / Weight	Day 5 Reps / Time / Weight
25	For time: - 35 air squats - 35 dumbbell push presses - 35 abmat sit-ups - 35 wall ball shots - 35 burpees - 35 med ball twists - 35 push-ups - 35 kettlebell swings - 35 dumbbell thrusters - 400 meter run					
26	20 Rounds for time: - 18 kettlebell swings - 6 goblet squats - 3 push-ups					
27	50-40-30-20-10 Reps for time: - double-unders - sit-ups					
28	10 Rounds for time: - 30 kettlebell swings - 30 burpees - 30 ghd sit-ups					
29	Every minute on the minute in 21 minutes: - minute 1: 20 push-ups - minute 2: 25 sit-ups - minute 3: 35 air squats repeat 7x					

Work-outs	Day 1 Reps / Time / Weight	Day 2 Reps / Time / Weight	Day 3 Reps / Time / Weight	Day 4 Reps / Time / Weight	Day 5 Reps / Time / Weight
30 For time: - 400-meter run - 30 wall-ball shots - 200-meter weighted run - 15 wall-ball shots - 400-meter run - 400-meter run - 30 wall-ball shots					
31 21-15-9-9-15-21 Reps for time: - deadlifts - burpees					
32 As many reps as possible in 20 minutes: - 10 push presses - 10 kettlebell swings - 15 box jumps					
33 For time: - 1 mile run - 31 push-ups then, 20 rounds of: - 3 deadlifts - 3 clean-and-jerks - 3 front squats then, perform: - 31 push-ups - 1 mile run					
34 4 Rounds for time: - 800 meter run - 50 push-ups - 50 sit-ups - 50 air squats					

	Day 1 Reps / Time / Weight	Day 2 Reps / Time / Weight	Day 3 Reps / Time / Weight	Day 4 Reps / Time / Weight	Day 5 Reps / Time / Weight
Work-outs					
35 For time: - 1 mile run - 21 clean-and-jerks - 800 meter run - 21 clean-and-jerks - 1 mile run					
36 For max reps of each: - 6 min. of double-under practice - 6 min. of clean and jerks - 3 min. of double-under practice - 3 min. of clean and jerks - 1 min. of double-under practice - 1 min. of clean and jerks					
37 Buy in: 15 devil presses then, 3 rounds of: - 8 burpees - 12 dumbbell snatches - 16 toes to bar cash out: 15 devil presses					
38 9 Rounds for time: - 9 hang power cleans - 9 front squats - 9 push presses - 9 burpees - 9 pull-ups - 9 dips - 9 box jumps - 9 sit-ups					

	Day 1 Reps / Time / Weight	Day 2 Reps / Time / Weight	Day 3 Reps / Time / Weight	Day 4 Reps / Time / Weight	Day 5 Reps / Time / Weight
Work-outs					
39	5 Rounds for time of: - row 500 m - 10 box jumps - 10 deadlifts - 10 wall-ball shots				
40	For time: - 150 double-unders - 15 meter single-arm overhead walking lunges - 25 alternating single-arm dumbbell thrusters - 15 meter single-arm overhead walking lunges - 25 alternating single-arm dumbbell thrusters - 15 meter single-arm overhead walking lunges - 150 double-unders time cap: 15 mins				
41	Run 2,500 meters				
42	5 Rounds for time: - 1000 meter row - 200 meter farmer carry - 50 meter waiter walk, right arm - 50 meter waiter walk, left arm				

Work-outs	Day 1 Reps / Time / Weight	Day 2 Reps / Time / Weight	Day 3 Reps / Time / Weight	Day 4 Reps / Time / Weight	Day 5 Reps / Time / Weight
43 For time: - 2,000 meter row then, complete as many reps as possible of in 20 min: - 5 toes-to-bars - 10 wall ball shots - 15 push-ups					
44 As many reps as possible in 25 minutes - 5 deadlifts - 5 hang power cleans - 5 front squats - 5 push press - 5 back squat					
45 For time: - 20 push-ups, 1 sit-up - 19 push-ups, 2 sit-ups - 18 push-ups, 3 sit-ups ...continue this pattern until... - 2 push-ups, 19 sit-ups - 1 push-up, 20 sit-ups					
46 For time: - 1 mile run - 100 calorie air bike - 100 calorie ski - 100 calorie row - 1 mile run					

Work-outs	Day 1 Reps / Time / Weight	Day 2 Reps / Time / Weight	Day 3 Reps / Time / Weight	Day 4 Reps / Time / Weight	Day 5 Reps / Time / Weight
47 As many reps as possible in 15 minutes: - 10 power cleans - 10 burpees over the bar - 20 deadlifts - 20 pull-ups					
48 Four 3-minute rounds of: - jog 100 meters with a medicine ball - max reps wall-ball shots rest 1 min. between rounds					
49 For time: 10-31-10-31 reps of: - wall ball shots - toes-to-bars - medball ball facing burpees after each round, complete: - 100 foot medball overhead walking lunges time cap: 25 minutes					

Work-outs	Day 1 Reps / Time / Weight	Day 2 Reps / Time / Weight	Day 3 Reps / Time / Weight	Day 4 Reps / Time / Weight	Day 5 Reps / Time / Weight
50 Two parts in 15 minutes: (15.1) as many reps as possible in 10 minutes: - 15 toes-to-bars - 10 deadlifts - 5 snatches then ("15.1a"), from 10:00-15:00 - 1-rep-max clean-and-jerk					
51 As many reps as possible in 12 minutes: - 1 minute of pull-ups - 3 minute of rowing - 1 minute of pull-ups - 2 minute of rowing - 1 minute of pull-ups - 3 minute of rowing - 1 minute of pull-ups					
52 As many reps as possible in 21 minutes: - 21 deadlifts - 21 wall ball shots - 21 toes-to-bars - 21 hand release push-ups					

Work-outs	Day 1 Reps / Time / Weight	Day 2 Reps / Time / Weight	Day 3 Reps / Time / Weight	Day 4 Reps / Time / Weight	Day 5 Reps / Time / Weight
53	5 Rounds for max reps: - hang power snatches - handstand push-ups rest as needed between rounds.				
54	6 rounds for time: - 20 calorie assault airbike - 15 air squats - 10 sit-ups				
55	For time: - 2,000 meter run - 50 pull-ups - 50 thrusters - 2,000 meter row				
56	150 reps for time, following the pattern: - 25 seconds of ring rows - 10 seconds of rest - 25 seconds of knee push-ups - 10 seconds of rest - 25 seconds of sit-ups - 10 seconds of rest - 25 seconds of squats - 10 seconds of rest				
57	6 Rounds for time: - 21 calorie row - 15 burpee box jump overs - 9 deadlifts				

Work-outs		Day 1 Reps / Time / Weight	Day 2 Reps / Time / Weight	Day 3 Reps / Time / Weight	Day 4 Reps / Time / Weight	Day 5 Reps / Time / Weight
58	For time: - 2000 meter row - 1 mile run - 2000 meter row time cap: 25 minutes					
59	For time: - 150 squats - 50 v-ups - 120 squats - 40 v-ups - 90 squats - 30 v-ups					
60	As many reps as possible in 21 minutes: - 400 meter run - 21 push-ups - 21 box jumps - 15 burpees - 9 pull-ups					
61	2 Rounds for time: - 10 devil presses - 400 meter run - 30 dumbbell sumo cleans - 300 meter run - 30 dumbbell floor presses - 200 meter run - 30 dumbbell front squats - 100 meter run - 10 devil presses rest 2 minutes					
62	5 Rounds for time: - 10 deadlifts - 50 foot single-arm dumbbell overhead walking lunges					

Work-outs	Day 1 Reps / Time / Weight	Day 2 Reps / Time / Weight	Day 3 Reps / Time / Weight	Day 4 Reps / Time / Weight	Day 5 Reps / Time / Weight
63 4 Rounds for time of: - run 200 meters - 20 kettlebell swings - 10 jumping pull-ups					
64 3 rounds for time of: - 50-ft. overhead walking lunge - 25 sit-ups					
65 3 Round for time: - 30 squat cleans - 30 pull-ups - 800 meter run					
66 For time: - 1 mile run - 45 box jump overs - 40 kettlebell swings - 35 burpees - 30 wall ball shots - 25 plate overhead lunges - 20 toes-to-bars - 15 kettlebell snatches - 10 pull-ups 1 mile run repeat back up the ladder to the top					
67 For time: - 50-meter broad jump - 25 alternating jumping lunges - 250-meter run					

	Day 1 Reps / Time / Weight	Day 2 Reps / Time / Weight	Day 3 Reps / Time / Weight	Day 4 Reps / Time / Weight	Day 5 Reps / Time / Weight
Work-outs					
68 As many reps as possible in 21 minutes - 10 devil presses - 20 alternating dumbbell lunges - 10 dumbbell push presses - 20 sit-ups					
69 For time: - 10 mile run - 150 burpee pull-ups					
70 5 Rounds for time: - 36 double-unders - 6 clusters - 1 rope climb *1 cluster is 1 clean and 1 thruster					
71 As many reps as possible in 11 minutes: - 5 deadlifts - 18 wall ball shots - 17 bar over burpees					
72 10 Rounds for time: - 4 clean-and-jerks - 4 bar over burpees					
73 4 Rounds for time of: - 10 overhead squats - 50 double-unders					
74 4 Rounds for time: - 400 meter run - 21 kettlebell swings - 12 pull-ups					

Work-outs	Day 1 Reps / Time / Weight	Day 2 Reps / Time / Weight	Day 3 Reps / Time / Weight	Day 4 Reps / Time / Weight	Day 5 Reps / Time / Weight
As many reps as possible in 18 minutes: - 80 double-unders - 10 wall ball shots - 8 deadlifts - 18 bar facing burpees - 10 wall ball shots					
four parts in 12 minutes every minute on the minute for 3 minutes: 15 dumbbell rows 10 push-ups every minute on the minute for 3 minutes: 10 dumbbell rows 10 push-ups every minute on the minute for 3 minutes: 5 dumbbell rows 10 push-ups then, as many reps as possible in 3 minutes: dumbbell rows					

Work-outs	Day 1 Reps / Time / Weight	Day 2 Reps / Time / Weight	Day 3 Reps / Time / Weight	Day 4 Reps / Time / Weight	Day 5 Reps / Time / Weight
77 For time: - 25 kettlebell swings - 25 wall ball shots - 25 overhead squats - 25 burpees - 25 lunges - 25 push jerks - 25 knees-to-elbows - 25 box jumps - 25 hang cleans - 25 sit-ups - 25 double-unders - 25 deadlifts					
78 For time: - 50 hang power snatches - 40 push presses - 50 sumo deadlift high pulls - 40 front squats					
79 4 Rounds for time of: - 400-meter row - 10 deadlifts - 20 box jumps					
80 6 Rounds for time: - 2 power snatches - 4 overhead squats - 6 overhead walking lunges					
81 As many reps as possible in 20 minutes: - 20 wall ball shots - 20 calorie row					

Work-outs	Day 1 Reps / Time / Weight	Day 2 Reps / Time / Weight	Day 3 Reps / Time / Weight	Day 4 Reps / Time / Weight	Day 5 Reps / Time / Weight
82 - 4 Rounds for time of: - 50-ft. dumbbell front-rack lunge - 15 pull-ups					
83 - 3 Rounds for time of: - 15 sit-ups - 30 squats - 45 single-unders					
84 - Complete as many rounds as possible in 10 minutes of: - 10 dumbbell deadlifts - 7 burpees - 4 dumbbell power cleans					
85 - As many reps as possible in 12 minutes: - 8 toes-to-bars - 8 dumbbell thrusters - 12 dumbbell walking lunges					
86 - As many reps as possible in 20 minutes: - 10 burpees - 30 deadlifts - 60 box jumps - 70 sit-ups					

		Day 1	Day 2	Day 3	Day 4	Day 5
	Work-outs	Reps / Time / Weight	Reps / Time / Weight	Reps / Time / Weight	Reps / Time / Weight	Reps / Time / Weight
87	5 Rounds for time of: - 25 kettlebell swings - 25 ghd sit-ups - 25 back extensions - 25 knees-to-elbows					
88	4 Rounds for time of: - run 400 meters - 4 rope climbs					
89	Complete as many rounds as possible in 7 minutes of: - 5 overhead squats - 5 box Jumps					
90	21-15-9 Reps for time: - cleans - ring dips					
91	4 Rounds for time of: - run 400 meters - 20 overhead squats					
92	As many reps as possible in 30 minutes: - 5 deadlifts - 13 push-ups - 9 box jumps					

Work-outs	Day 1 Reps / Time / Weight	Day 2 Reps / Time / Weight	Day 3 Reps / Time / Weight	Day 4 Reps / Time / Weight	Day 5 Reps / Time / Weight
93. As many reps as possible in 7 minutes: - 1 pull-up - 2 push presses - 2 pull-ups - 4 push presses continue with this pattern, adding 1 pull-up and 2 push presses each round.					
94. 3 Rounds for total reps in 20 minutes - 1 minute wall ball shots - 1 minute sumo deadlift high-pulls - 1 minute box jumps - 1 minute push press - 1 minute row - 1 minute rest					
95. For time: - 25 wall ball shots - 25 pull-ups - 50 sit-ups - 50 air squats - 100 push-ups - 20 calorie air bike - 100 kettlebell swings					
96. Complete as many rounds as possible in 12 minutes of: - 1 squat snatch - 3 clean and jerks - 30 double-unders					

Work-outs	Day 1 Reps / Time / Weight	Day 2 Reps / Time / Weight	Day 3 Reps / Time / Weight	Day 4 Reps / Time / Weight	Day 5 Reps / Time / Weight
97	10 Rounds for time: - 10 kettlebell thrusters - 15 kettlebell sumo deadlift high-pulls - 10 burpee box jumps - 15 calorie assault air bike					
98	For time: - 40 kettlebell swings - run 800 meters - 40 kettlebell swings					
99	5 Rounds for time: - 15 dumbbell deadlifts - 9 pull-ups - 3 curtis p - rest two minutes - 5 rounds - 20 dumbbell overhead lunge (alternating lunge) - 10 toes to bar - 5 man makers finisher 5 minute cardio of choice					
100	11 Rounds for time: - 11 mountain climbers - 11 air squats - 11 hand release push-ups - 11 box jump burpees - 200 meter run					

Work-outs	Day 1 Reps / Time / Weight	Day 2 Reps / Time / Weight	Day 3 Reps / Time / Weight	Day 4 Reps / Time / Weight	Day 5 Reps / Time / Weight
101 10 Rounds for time: - 5 squat cleans - 10 burpee box jumps					
102 70-40-10 Reps for time: - burpees - push-ups - sit-ups - air squats					
103 For max reps in 25 mins: - max burpee box jump-overs rest 5 mins - max 10 min shuttle runs rest 4 mins - max power cleans rest 3 mins - max wall ball shots rest 2 mins - max unbroken pull-ups					
104 8 Rounds for time: - 400 meter run - 20 back squats					
105 For time: - row 500 meters - 25 sit-ups - row 750 meters - 20 sit-ups - row 1,000 meters - 15 sit-ups					
106 10 Rounds for time of: - 30 seconds of l-sit, unbroken - 10 box jumps					

Work-outs	Day 1 Reps / Time / Weight	Day 2 Reps / Time / Weight	Day 3 Reps / Time / Weight	Day 4 Reps / Time / Weight	Day 5 Reps / Time / Weight
107 5 Rounds for time of: - 1-minute plank hold - 21 sit-ups					
108 Complete as many rounds as possible in 20 minutes of: - 3 rope climbs, lying to standing - 20 squats - 40 single-unders					
109 For time: - 25 pull-ups - 50 deadlifts - 50 push-ups - 50 box jumps - 50 floor wipers - 50 alternating kettlebell clean-and-presses - 25 pull-ups					
110 For time: - 1,500-meter row then, 5 rounds of: - 10 bar muscle-ups - 7 push jerks					
111 As many reps as possible in 18 minutes: - 13 hang power snatches - 13 burpees - 13 thrusters - 13 pull-ups					

Work-outs	Day 1 Reps / Time / Weight	Day 2 Reps / Time / Weight	Day 3 Reps / Time / Weight	Day 4 Reps / Time / Weight	Day 5 Reps / Time / Weight
3 Rounds for time: - 12 burpees - 12 thrusters - 12 burpees - 12 power snatches - 12 burpees - 12 push jerks - 12 burpees - 12 hang squat cleans - 12 burpees - 12 overhead squats					
For time: - 50 walking lunges - 25 chest-to-bar pull-ups - 50 box jumps - 25 triple-unders - 50 back extensions - 25 ring dips - 50 knees-to-elbows - 25 wall ball - 50 sit-ups - 5 rope climbs					
For time: - 100 deadlifts - 100 power cleans - 100 ground-to-overheads - 45 burpees					

Work-outs	Day 1 Reps / Time / Weight	Day 2 Reps / Time / Weight	Day 3 Reps / Time / Weight	Day 4 Reps / Time / Weight	Day 5 Reps / Time / Weight
As many reps as possible in 20 minutes: - 40 burpees - 30 snatches - 30 burpees - 30 snatches - 20 burpees - 30 snatches 10 burpees max snatches					
For time: 30 burpees - 20 sit-ups - 25 push-ups - 30 tuck jumps - 20 squats - 30 jumping jacks - 20 lunges - 30 crunches					
21-17-13 Reps for time of: - cleans - push-ups					
For time: - 100 burpee pull-ups					
Every other minute on the minute for 20 minutes: - 30 double-unders - max push-up + renegade rows					

Work-outs	Day 1 Reps / Time / Weight	Day 2 Reps / Time / Weight	Day 3 Reps / Time / Weight	Day 4 Reps / Time / Weight	Day 5 Reps / Time / Weight
As many reps as possible in 20 minutes: - 5 deadlifts - 10 burpee pull-ups - 10 kettlebell swings - 200 meter run					
As many reps as possible in 21 minutes: - 7 squat cleans - 7 push press - 7 back squats - 200 meter run					
4 Rounds for time of: - run 200 m - 25 walking lunges					
5 Rounds for time: - 15 calorie assault bike - 10 burpees					
3 Rounds for time of: - run 500 meters - 30 deadlifts					
Complete as many rounds as possible in 10 minutes of: - 5 power snatches - 10 overhead walking lunges - 1 rope climb					

Work-outs	Day 1 Reps / Time / Weight	Day 2 Reps / Time / Weight	Day 3 Reps / Time / Weight	Day 4 Reps / Time / Weight	Day 5 Reps / Time / Weight
Complete as many rounds as possible in 15 minutes of: - 15 hanging knee raises - 25-calorie row - 40 knee push-ups - 25 box jumps - 15 pull-ups					
For time: - 40 box jumps - 40 jumping pull-ups - 40 kettlebell swings - 40 walking-lunge steps - 40 knees-to-elbows - 40 push presses - 40 back extensions - 40 wall-ball shots - 40 burpees - 40 double-unders					

Work-outs	Day 1 Reps / Time / Weight	Day 2 Reps / Time / Weight	Day 3 Reps / Time / Weight	Day 4 Reps / Time / Weight	Day 5 Reps / Time / Weight
As many reps as possible in 26 minutes: - 31 double-unders - 25 pull-ups - 23 push-ups - 23 air squats - 23 abmat sit-ups - 22 kettlebell swings 128 - 22 calorie row - 22 toes-to-bars - 20 wall ball shots - 20 box jumps - 20 alternating dumbbell snatches - 20 burpees - 20 dumbbell thrusters cash-out: 3 minute plank hold					
For time: - 10 tabata air squats 129 - 20 snatches - 10 tabata push-ups - 20 thrusters					
30 Rounds for time: - 6 wall ball shots 130 - 4 handstand push-ups - 2 power clean					
5 Rounds for time: - 10 deadlifts 131 - 50 foot single-arm dumbbell overhead walking lunges					

Work-outs	Day 1 Reps / Time / Weight	Day 2 Reps / Time / Weight	Day 3 Reps / Time / Weight	Day 4 Reps / Time / Weight	Day 5 Reps / Time / Weight
For time: - 1 wall walk - 10 double-unders - 3 wall walks - 30 double-unders - 6 wall walks 132 - 60 double-unders - 9 wall walks - 90 double-unders - 15 wall walks - 150 double-unders - 21 wall walks - 210 double-unders					
5 Rounds of - 15 bench presses 133 - 15 bent over rows - 12 skull crushers - 12 bicep curls					
For time: - 10 overhead squats - 10 box jump-overs - 10 thrusters - 10 power cleans - 10 toes-to-bars 134 - 10 burpee muscle-ups - 10 toes-to-bars - 10 power cleans - 10 thrusters - 10 box jump-overs - 10 overhead squats					
Complete as many rounds as possible in 15 minutes of: 135 - row 25 calories - 25 ghd sit-ups - 15 box jumps					

Work-outs	Day 1 Reps / Time / Weight	Day 2 Reps / Time / Weight	Day 3 Reps / Time / Weight	Day 4 Reps / Time / Weight	Day 5 Reps / Time / Weight
136 For time: - row 300 meters - 30 bench presses - row 400 meters - 20 bench presses - row 500 meters - 10 bench presses					
137 5 Rounds for time: - 15 calorie assault bike - 10 burpees					
138 Complete as many rounds as possible in 20 minutes of: - 30-second seated leg raises - 15 elevated push-ups - 60 single-unders					
139 10 Rounds for time of: - 8 ground-to-overheads - 10 bar-facing burpees					
140 For time: - 1,000 meter row - 25 clean-and-jerks - 1,000 meter row - 50 burpees - 1,000 meter row - 75 wall ball shots					
141 Row 5,000 meters					
142 5 Rounds of: - 20 pull-ups - 30 push-ups - 40 sit-ups - 50 squats					

Work-outs	Day 1 Reps / Time / Weight	Day 2 Reps / Time / Weight	Day 3 Reps / Time / Weight	Day 4 Reps / Time / Weight	Day 5 Reps / Time / Weight
For time: - 60 squats - 30 sit-ups - 40 squats - 20 sit-ups - 20 squats - 10 sit-ups					
For time: - 400 meter run - 22 snatches - 22 pull-ups - 22 medicine ball cleans - 22 elbow plank to push-ups - 22 wall ball shots - 22 deadlifts - 22 air squats - 22 overhead walking lunges - 22 box jumps - 22 power cleans - 4x20 second bar hang - 22 calorie row - 22 handstand push-ups - 22 back squats - 22 chest-to-bar pull-ups - 22 bar facing burpees - 22 thrusters - 22 jerks - 2 rope climbs - 22 overhead squats - 22 kettlebell swings					

Work-outs	Day 1 Reps / Time / Weight	Day 2 Reps / Time / Weight	Day 3 Reps / Time / Weight	Day 4 Reps / Time / Weight	Day 5 Reps / Time / Weight
145 For time: - 50 deadlifts - 50 double kettlebell swings - 50 push-ups - 50 clean-and-jerks - 50 pull-ups - 50 kettlebell taters - 50 box jumps - 50 wall climbs - 50 knee-to-elbows - 50 double-unders					
146 5 Rounds for time: - 500 meter run - 15 overhead squats - 15 bar facing burpees					
147 Complete as many reps in 12 minutes of: - jump touch burpees					
148 As many reps as possible in 25 minutes - 5 handstand push-ups - 10 pistols (alternating legs) - 15 pull-ups					
149 Complete as many rounds as possible in 10 minutes of: - 50 single-unders - 100-m farmers carry					

Work-outs	Day 1 Reps / Time / Weight	Day 2 Reps / Time / Weight	Day 3 Reps / Time / Weight	Day 4 Reps / Time / Weight	Day 5 Reps / Time / Weight
150 5 Rounds for time of: - 3 power cleans - 60-yard shuttle sprint					
151 8 Rounds for time: - 10 man makers - 20 dumbbell deadlifts - 30 single-arm dumbbell snatches (15 per side) - 40 single-arm overhead lunges (20 per side) - 50 dumbbell swings use one pair of dumbbells throughout					
152 Complete as many rounds as possible in 25 minutes of: - 5 jumping chest-to-bar pull-ups - 10 knee push-ups - 20 walking lunges *after every 3 rounds, run 500 meters					
153 8 Rounds of: - 1 minute of rowing rest 15 seconds - 30 seconds of push-ups rest 15 seconds					

Work-outs	Day 1 Reps / Time / Weight	Day 2 Reps / Time / Weight	Day 3 Reps / Time / Weight	Day 4 Reps / Time / Weight	Day 5 Reps / Time / Weight
154 4 Rounds for time of: - 21 thrusters - 21 assisted pull-ups					
155 As many reps as possible in 25 minutes: - 1 rope climb - 6 pull-ups - 6 front squats - 4 shoulder-to-overheads					
156 4 Rounds for time of: - 15 dumbbell push jerks - 50 single-unders - 15 step-ups - 50 single-unders					
157 5 Rounds for time: - 25 handstand push-ups - 35 deadlifts - 45 sit-ups - 55 double-unders					
158 For time: - 500-m row - 50 assisted pull-ups - 35-ft. walking lunge, weight back-racked - 35-ft. walking lunge, weight front-racked - 35-ft. walking lunge, weight overhead					

Work-outs	Day 1 Reps / Time / Weight	Day 2 Reps / Time / Weight	Day 3 Reps / Time / Weight	Day 4 Reps / Time / Weight	Day 5 Reps / Time / Weight
159 35 snatches for time					
160 5 Rounds for time: - 20 air squats - 20 alternating lunges - 20 alternating split squat jumps - 15 squat jumps					
161 7 Rounds for time: - 10 back squats - 1,000 meter row					
162 21-15-9 Reps for time: - kettlebell swings - burpees					
163 4 Rounds for time of: - run 600 meters - rest 2 minutes					
164 4 Rounds for time: - 6 left-hand turkish get-ups - 6 right-hand turkish get-ups - 4 rope climbs, lying to standing					
165 As many reps as possible in 20 minutes: - 20 calorie ski erg - 20 sandbag lunges - 20 burpee broad jumps					

Work-outs	Day 1 Reps / Time / Weight	Day 2 Reps / Time / Weight	Day 3 Reps / Time / Weight	Day 4 Reps / Time / Weight	Day 5 Reps / Time / Weight
166 Every minute on the minute for 20 minutes - odd minutes: 24 calorie assault bike - even minutes: 18 ghd sit-ups					
167 5 Rounds for time - 400 meter run - 40 box jumps - 40 wall ball shots					
168 3 Rounds of: - 5 minutes of rowing 1 minutes of rest					
169 For time: - 100 calorie row - 100 calorie ski erg - 100 calorie assault air bike every 2 minutes, perform: - 7 burpees					
170 5 Rounds for time of: - row 500 meters - 7 thrusters					
171 7 Rounds for time: - 15 kettlebell swings - 15 power cleans - 15 box jumps					
172 Complete as many rounds as possible in 18 minutes of: - 15 box jumps - 12 push presses - 9 toes-to-bars					

Work-outs	Day 1 Reps / Time / Weight	Day 2 Reps / Time / Weight	Day 3 Reps / Time / Weight	Day 4 Reps / Time / Weight	Day 5 Reps / Time / Weight
For time: - row 350 meters - 20 push presses - row 350 meters - 15 push presses - row 350 meters - 10 push presses - row 350 meters - 5 push presses					
For time: - 500-meter row - 20 pull-ups - 10 overhead squats, with a dowel - 10 pull-ups - 20 overhead squats, with a dowel - 10 pull-ups - 30 overhead squats, with a dowel - 500-meter row					
As many reps as possible in 25 minutes: - 10 pull-ups - 12 push presses - 10 box jumps - 12 kettlebell swings - 10 toes-to-bars - 12 power cleans - 10 burpees					

	Day 1 Reps / Time / Weight	Day 2 Reps / Time / Weight	Day 3 Reps / Time / Weight	Day 4 Reps / Time / Weight	Day 5 Reps / Time / Weight
Work-outs					
176 For time: 13-12-11-10-9-8-7-6-5-4-3-2-1 reps of: - hand release push-ups - air squats - sit ups					
177 4 Rounds, each for time, of: - 25 knee push-ups - 25 deadlifts - 25 sit-ups - 50 single-unders					
178 For time: - 100 thrusters - 10 burpees to start and at the top of every minute					
179 Complete as many rounds as possible in 12 minutes of: - 6 power cleans - 12 hanging knee-raises					
180 As many reps as possible in 25 minutes: - 5 renegade rows - 10 burpee box jump over - 15 abmat sit ups - 20 dual db overhead walking lunges - 25 double-unders					

Work-outs	Day 1 Reps / Time / Weight	Day 2 Reps / Time / Weight	Day 3 Reps / Time / Weight	Day 4 Reps / Time / Weight	Day 5 Reps / Time / Weight
181 Complete as many rounds as possible in 20 minutes of: - 400 meter run - 10 pull-ups - 10 ring dips					
182 Complete as many rounds as possible in 12 minutes of: - 4 shoulder presses - 8 sumo deadlift high pulls - 12 front squats					
183 Run 2 mile					
184 For time: - 10 handstand push-ups - 15 deadlifts - 25 box jumps - 50 pull-ups - 100 wall ball shots - 200 double-unders - 400 meter run					
185 6 Rounds for time of: - 6 front squats - 6 push-ups					
186 For time: - 30 kettlebell swings - 200-meter run - 25 kettlebell swings - 400-meter run - 20 kettlebell swings - 800-meter run - 10 kettlebell swings					

Work-outs	Day 1 Reps / Time / Weight	Day 2 Reps / Time / Weight	Day 3 Reps / Time / Weight	Day 4 Reps / Time / Weight	Day 5 Reps / Time / Weight
For time: - 60 power snatches					
For time: - 10 overhead squats - 10 box jump overs - 10 fat bar thrusters - 10 power cleans - 10 toes-to-bars - 10 burpee muscle-ups - 10 toes-to-bars - 10 power cleans - 10 fat bar thrusters - 10 box jump overs - 10 overhead squats time cap: 15 mins					
As many reps as possible in 30 minutes: - 15 hang power cleans - 15 bar facing burpees - 1,000 meter bike - 15 sumo deadlift high pulls - 15 strict ring dips					
11 Rounds for time: - 11 burpees - 11 air squats - 11 push-ups - 11 sit-ups time cap: 30 minutes					

Work-outs	Day 1 Reps / Time / Weight	Day 2 Reps / Time / Weight	Day 3 Reps / Time / Weight	Day 4 Reps / Time / Weight	Day 5 Reps / Time / Weight
191 Every minute on the minute for 25 minutes perform: - 4 jumping pull-ups - 7 knee push-ups - 10 squats					
192 For time: - 30 box jumps - 30 jumping pull-ups - 30 kettlebell swings - 30 lunges - 30 knees-to-elbows - 30 push presses - 30 back extensions - 30 wall ball shots - 30 burpees - 30 double-unders time cap: 30 minutes					
193 3 Rounds for time of: - run 400 meters - 15 ring rows - 20 push-ups - 25 squats					
194 For time: - back squat 9-9-9 reps - shoulder press 9-9-9 reps - deadlift 9-9-9 reps					
195 For time: - 1,000 meter row - 50 thrusters - 25 pull-ups					

Work-outs	Day 1 Reps / Time / Weight	Day 2 Reps / Time / Weight	Day 3 Reps / Time / Weight	Day 4 Reps / Time / Weight	Day 5 Reps / Time / Weight
196 6 Rounds for time: - 12 deadlifts - 9 hang power cleans - 6 push jerks					
197 As many reps as possible in 21 minutes: - 50 wall ball shots - 50 double-unders - 40 box jumps - 40 toes-to-bars - 30 chest-to-bar pull-ups - 30 burpees - 20 power cleans - 20 jerks - 10 power snatches - 10 muscle-ups					
198 20 Rounds for time: - 6 strict pull-ups - 20 push-ups					
199 As many repetitions as possible in 5 rounds of: - max bench press - max pull-ups					
200 Complete as many rounds as possible in 12 minutes of: - 12 abmat sit-ups - 12 walking lunges - 24-yard waiter walk					
201 30-20-10 Reps for time of: - row (calories) - wall-ball shots					

Work-outs	Day 1 Reps / Time / Weight	Day 2 Reps / Time / Weight	Day 3 Reps / Time / Weight	Day 4 Reps / Time / Weight	Day 5 Reps / Time / Weight
For time: - 20 weighted lunge steps - 20 muscle-ups - 200-ft. handstand walk 202 - 20 hang power cleans - 20 box jumps - 20 deficit handstand push-ups - 20 front squats					
203 For time: - 40 clean-and-jerks					
As many reps as possible in 25 minutes: 204 - 12 chest-to-bar pull-ups - 2 deadlifts - 10 handstand push-ups					
6 Rounds for time: 205 - 20 kettlebell swings - 400 meter run					
3 Rounds for time of: 206 - row 250 meters - run 250 meters - 25 sit-ups					
For time: - muscle snatch 1-1-1-1-1 reps 207 - power snatch 1-1-1-1-1 reps - squat snatch 1-1-1-1-1 reps					

Work-outs	Day 1 Reps / Time / Weight	Day 2 Reps / Time / Weight	Day 3 Reps / Time / Weight	Day 4 Reps / Time / Weight	Day 5 Reps / Time / Weight
208 As many reps as possible in 20 minutes - 500 meter run - max pull-ups					
209 Cash-in: 1,000 meter run as many reps as possible in 22 minutes of: - 21 air squats - 7 burpees - 14 push-ups cash-out: 1,000 meter run					
210 Complete as many rounds as possible in 15 minutes of: - 5 strict toes-to-bars - 10 ghd sit-ups - 15 hip extensions					
211 As many reps as possible in 33 minutes: 2 rounds of: - 3 man makers - 20 kettlebell swings - 100 single-unders rest 3 minutes in the remaining time, as many reps as possible of: - 800 meter run - 30 wall ball shots - 20 calorie row - 10 burpees					

Work-outs	Day 1 Reps / Time / Weight	Day 2 Reps / Time / Weight	Day 3 Reps / Time / Weight	Day 4 Reps / Time / Weight	Day 5 Reps / Time / Weight
212 For time: - 100 sandbag cleans over the shoulder every 90 seconds perform: - 5 strict pull-ups					
213 Complete as many burpees as possible in 10 minutes					
214 As many reps as possible in 12 minutes: - 3 thrusters - 3 chest-to-bar pull-ups - 6 thrusters - 6 chest-to-bar pull-ups - 9 thrusters - 9 chest-to-bar pull-ups if you complete the round of 9, complete a round of 12, then go on to 15, etc.					
215 10 Rounds for time: - 10 ground-to-overheads - 10 bar facing burpees time cap: 15 minutes					

Work-outs	Day 1 Reps / Time / Weight	Day 2 Reps / Time / Weight	Day 3 Reps / Time / Weight	Day 4 Reps / Time / Weight	Day 5 Reps / Time / Weight
216 As many reps as possible in 15 minutes: - 5 shoulder-to-overheads - 10 deadlifts - 15 box jumps					
217 For time: - 20 knee raises - 1-mile run - 20 knee raises - 1-mile run - 20 knee raises					
218 For time: - 40 muscle-ups - 80-cal. row - 120 wall-ball shots					
219 As many reps as possible in 14 minutes: - 60 calorie row - 50 toes-to-bars - 40 wall ball shots - 30 cleans - 20 muscle-ups					
220 As many reps as possible in 15 minutes: - 5 burpees - 10 push-ups - 15 air squats - 6 meter bear crawl (3 meter there and back)					

Work-outs	Day 1 Reps / Time / Weight	Day 2 Reps / Time / Weight	Day 3 Reps / Time / Weight	Day 4 Reps / Time / Weight	Day 5 Reps / Time / Weight
221 For total reps: - 3 sets of shoulder presses, empty barbell - 3 sets of assisted pull-ups - 3 sets of push presses, empty barbell - 3 sets of assisted pull-ups - 3 sets of push jerks, empty barbell - 3 sets of assisted pull-ups rest 30 sec. between sets.					
222 As many reps as possible in 10 minutes: - 3 squat cleans - 2 jerks					
223 For time: - 20 single-leg squat, alternating - 20-yard handstand walk - 30 single-leg squat, alternating - 30-yard handstand walk - 40 single-leg squat, alternating - 40-yard handstand walk - 50 single-leg squat, alternating - 50-yard handstand walk					

	Day 1	Day 2	Day 3	Day 4	Day 5
Work-outs	**Reps / Time / Weight**	**Reps / Time / Weight**	**Reps / Time / Weight**	**Reps / Time / Weight**	**Reps / Time / Weight**
5 Rounds for time: - 20 pull-ups - 30 push-ups - 40 sit-ups - 50 air squats 2 minutes rest					
Complete as much as possible in 15 minutes of: - 1 jumping pull-up + 1 assisted push-ups - 5 medicine-ball cleans - 2 jumping pull-up + 2 assisted push-ups - 10 medicine-ball cleans - 3 jumping pull-up + 3 assisted push-ups - 15 medicine-ball cleans - 4 jumping pull-up + 4 assisted push-ups - 20 medicine-ball cleans					
For time: - 30 pull-ups - 50 wall ball shots - 50 sit-ups - 100 kettlebell swings perform every two minutes: - 10 burpees					

Work-outs	Day 1 Reps / Time / Weight	Day 2 Reps / Time / Weight	Day 3 Reps / Time / Weight	Day 4 Reps / Time / Weight	Day 5 Reps / Time / Weight
For time: - 10 dumbbell snatches - 15 burpee box jump overs - 20 dumbbell snatches - 15 burpee box jump overs - 30 dumbbell snatches 227 - 15 burpee box jump overs - 40 dumbbell snatches - 15 burpee box jump overs - 50 dumbbell snatches - 15 burpee box jump overs time cap: 25 minutes					
9-7-5 Reps for time: 228 - muscle-ups - squat snatches					
5 Rounds for time: - 3 rope climbs 229 - 11 toes-to-bars - 21 overhead walking lunges - 400 meter run					
5 Rounds for time of: 230 - lunge 50 meters - run 150 meters					

Work-outs	Day 1 Reps / Time / Weight	Day 2 Reps / Time / Weight	Day 3 Reps / Time / Weight	Day 4 Reps / Time / Weight	Day 5 Reps / Time / Weight
231 For time: - 40 ring rows - 40 knee push-ups - 40 sit-ups - 40 squats					
232 21-15-9 Reps for time: - handstand push-ups - ring dips - push-ups					
233 3 Rounds for time: - 500 meter row - 25 deadlifts - 25 box jumps					
234 For time: - 50 wall ball shots - 45 deadlifts - 40 hand release push-ups - 35 box jumps - 30 toes-to-bars - 25 burpees - 20 power cleans - 15 push presses - 10 weighted lunges - 5 thrusters					
235 For time: - run 1,500 meters rest 3 minutes - run 1,000 meters rest 2 minute - run 500 meters					

Work-outs	Day 1 Reps / Time / Weight	Day 2 Reps / Time / Weight	Day 3 Reps / Time / Weight	Day 4 Reps / Time / Weight	Day 5 Reps / Time / Weight
For time: - 40 wall ball shots - 30 hang cleans - 40 pull-ups - 30 deadlifts - 40 push-ups - 30 box jumps - 40 kettlebell swings - 30 toes-to-bars - 40 air squats - 30 hang snatches - 40 double-unders - 30 sit-ups - 40 burpees 300 meter run at start and after each 40-rep movement					
For time - 25 deadlifts - 500 meter run - 25 kettlebell swings - 500 meter run - 25 overhead squats - 500 meter run - 25 burpees - 500 meter run - 25 chest-to-bar pull-ups - 500 meter run - 25 box jumps - 500 meter run - 25 dumbbell squat cleans - 500 meter run					

Work-outs	Day 1 Reps / Time / Weight	Day 2 Reps / Time / Weight	Day 3 Reps / Time / Weight	Day 4 Reps / Time / Weight	Day 5 Reps / Time / Weight
238 For time: - 10 thrusters - 15 bar-facing burpees - 20 thrusters - 25 bar-facing burpees - 30 thrusters - 35 bar-facing burpees					
239 5 Rounds: - 10 hang power snatches - 10 push-ups					
240 For time: - 30 clean-and-jerks - 1 mile run - 10 rope climbs - 1 mile run - 100 burpees					
241 As many reps as possible in 20 minutes: - 6 dumbbell man makers - 7 box step ups					
242 21-15-9 Reps for time of: - push-up - pull-up					

Work-outs	Day 1 Reps / Time / Weight	Day 2 Reps / Time / Weight	Day 3 Reps / Time / Weight	Day 4 Reps / Time / Weight	Day 5 Reps / Time / Weight
243 As many reps as possible in 30 minutes 2 rounds of: - 4 man makers - 20 kettlebell swings - 80 single-unders rest 3 minutes in the remaining time, as many reps as possible of: - 800 meter run - 30 wall ball shots - 20 calorie row - 10 burpees					
244 35 Clean and jerks for time					
245 Five rounds of as many reps as possibles in 24 minutes: as many reps as possible in 4 minutes per round - 3 power cleans - 6 push-ups - 9 air squats - 12 deadlifts 1 minute rest, then repeat (5 times total)					
246 27-21-15-9 Reps for time of: - squat cleans - ring dips					

Work-outs	Day 1 Reps / Time / Weight	Day 2 Reps / Time / Weight	Day 3 Reps / Time / Weight	Day 4 Reps / Time / Weight	Day 5 Reps / Time / Weight
247 4 Rounds for time of: - 15 push-ups - 15 ring dips - 1,000-meter row					
248 15-12-9 Reps: - clean-and-jerks					
249 As many reps as possible in 12 minutes: - 2 minute burpees 2 minute rest - tabata sit-up 2 minute rest - 2 minute jumping jacks					
250 As many reps as possible in 15 minutes: - 8 power cleans - 8 overhead presses - 10 high-five push-ups					
251 For time: - 20 pull-ups + 20 push-ups - 20-meter lunge - 200 single-unders - 10 pull-ups + 10 push-ups - 20-meter lunge - 100 single-unders - 5 pull-ups + 5 push-ups - 10-meter lunge - 60 single-unders					

	Day 1	Day 2	Day 3	Day 4	Day 5
Work-outs	Reps / Time / Weight	Reps / Time / Weight	Reps / Time / Weight	Reps / Time / Weight	Reps / Time / Weight
252 For time: - 21 dumbbell thrusters - 400 meter run - 15 dumbbell thrusters - 400 meter run - 9 dumbbell thrusters - 400 meter run					
253 For time: - 3,000 meter row - 300 double-unders - 2 mile run					
254 Complete as many rounds as possible in 20 minutes of: - 5 power cleans - 5 front squats - 5 push presses - 20 burpees					
255 As many reps as possible 12: - 3 cleans - 250 meter row					
256 Complete as many rounds as possible in 18 minutes of: - 15 ox jumps - 12 push presses - 9 toes-to-bar					

Work-outs	Day 1 Reps / Time / Weight	Day 2 Reps / Time / Weight	Day 3 Reps / Time / Weight	Day 4 Reps / Time / Weight	Day 5 Reps / Time / Weight
For time: - 2 rope climbs, lying to standing - 30 squats, alternating - 30 dumbbell snatches, alternating - 2 rope climbs, lying to standing - 20 squats, alternating - 20 dumbbell snatches, alternating - 2 rope climb, lying to standing - 10 squats, alternating - 10 dumbbell snatches, alternating - 2 rope climb, lying to standing - 5 squats, alternating - 5 dumbbell snatches, alternating					

257

Work-outs	Day 1 Reps / Time / Weight	Day 2 Reps / Time / Weight	Day 3 Reps / Time / Weight	Day 4 Reps / Time / Weight	Day 5 Reps / Time / Weight
3 Rounds of: - 10 push-ups - 10 dumbbell hang power cleans - 50 single-unders rest 1 min., then: 3 rounds of: - 10 knee push-ups - 10 dumbbell shoulder-to-overheads - 50 single-unders					
As many reps as possible in 13 minutes: 2 rounds of: - 50 ft dumbbell walking lunges - 16 toe-to-bars - 8 dumbbell power cleans then, 2 rounds of: - 50 ft dumbbell walking lunges - 16 bar muscle-ups - 8 dumbbell power cleans					
3 Rounds for time of: - 40 pull-ups - 400-meter run					
11 Rounds of: - 1 minute of burpees - 1 minute of air squats - 1 minute of double unders 1 minute rest					

Work-outs	Day 1 Reps / Time / Weight	Day 2 Reps / Time / Weight	Day 3 Reps / Time / Weight	Day 4 Reps / Time / Weight	Day 5 Reps / Time / Weight
As many reps as possible in 10 minutes: - 1 pull-up - 2 push presses - 2 pull-ups - 4 push presses continue with this pattern, adding 1 pull-up and 2 push presses each round					
As many reps as possible in 21 minutes: - 10 pull-ups - 20 push-ups - 30 air squats - 15 pull-ups - 30 push-ups - 45 air squats - 20 pull-ups - 40 push-ups - 60 air squats - 25 pull-ups - 50 push-ups - 75 air squats - 30 pull-ups - 60 push-ups - 90 air squats					
For time: - 21 dumbbell thrusters - 400 meter run - 18 dumbbell thrusters - 400 meter run - 15 dumbbell thrusters - 400 meter run					

Work-outs	Day 1 Reps / Time / Weight	Day 2 Reps / Time / Weight	Day 3 Reps / Time / Weight	Day 4 Reps / Time / Weight	Day 5 Reps / Time / Weight
5 Rounds for time of: - run 800 meters - 25 overhead squats - 25 sumo deadlift high pulls					
10 Rounds for time: - 20 push-ups - 20 air squats - 20 mountain climbers (left+right=1) - 20 jumping jacks					
For time: - 10 dumbbell snatches - 15 burpee box jump-overs - 20 dumbbell snatches - 15 burpee box jump-overs - 30 dumbbell snatches - 15 burpee box jump-overs - 40 dumbbell snatches - 15 burpee box jump-overs - 50 dumbbell snatches - 15 burpee box jump-overs					

Work-outs	Day 1 Reps / Time / Weight	Day 2 Reps / Time / Weight	Day 3 Reps / Time / Weight	Day 4 Reps / Time / Weight	Day 5 Reps / Time / Weight
For time: - 10 burpees - 25 push-ups - 10 burpees - 25 push-ups - 50 lunges - 10 burpees 268 - 25 push-ups - 50 lunges - 100 sit-ups - 10 burpees - 25 push-ups - 50 lunges - 100 sit-ups - 150 air squats					
6 Rounds for total reps in 24 minutes: - 1 minute of rowing - 1 minute of 269 burpees - 1 minute of double-unders - 1 minute rest					
For time: - 100 pull-ups 270 - 100 push-ups - 100 sit-ups - 100 air squats					
30-20-10-5 Reps for time: 271 - row (calories) - thrusters					
As many reps as possible in 20 minutes: 272 - 20 overhead squats - 20 back squats - 400 meter run					

Work-outs	Day 1 Reps / Time / Weight	Day 2 Reps / Time / Weight	Day 3 Reps / Time / Weight	Day 4 Reps / Time / Weight	Day 5 Reps / Time / Weight
273 Complete as many rounds as possible in 20 minutes of: - 400 meter run - 50 double-unders - 15 toes-to-bars					
274 For time: - 100 dumbbell hang clean thrusters - 5 burpees to start, and at the top of each minute					
275 3 Rounds for time of: - run 200 meters - 20 hanging knee raises - run 200 meters - 20 dumbbell thrusters					
276 21-7-11 Reps for time - burpees - kettlebell swings - double-unders					
277 5 Rounds for time: - 15 hollow rocks - 15 v-ups - 15 tuck ups - 15 second hollow hold 1 minute rest					
278 For time: - 150 wall ball shots					

Work-outs	Day 1 Reps / Time / Weight	Day 2 Reps / Time / Weight	Day 3 Reps / Time / Weight	Day 4 Reps / Time / Weight	Day 5 Reps / Time / Weight
279 As many reps as possible in 20 minutes: - 7 pull-ups - 11 push-ups - 15 air squats					
280 As many reps as possible in 20 minutes: - 1 mile run then, 5 rounds of: - 30 air squats - 20 push-ups if you finish, start again on the run.					
281 Buy in: 15 devil presses then, 3 rounds of: - 8 burpees - 12 dumbbell snatches - 16 toes to bar cash out: 15 devil presses					
282 For time: - 100 kettlebell swings - 100 sit-ups - 100 air squats - 100 push-ups					
283 For time: - row 2,000 meters - 100 wall-ball shots - 20 muscle-ups					

	Day 1 Reps / Time / Weight	Day 2 Reps / Time / Weight	Day 3 Reps / Time / Weight	Day 4 Reps / Time / Weight	Day 5 Reps / Time / Weight
Work-outs					
284 As many reps as possible in 20 minutes: - 80 double-unders - 10 wall ball shots - 10 deadlifts - 10 bar facing burpees - 10 wall ball shots					
285 21-15-9 Reps for time: - deadlifts - handstand push-ups					
286 5 2-minute rounds of: - 20 dumbbell box step-ups - max reps of dumbbell push presses rest 2 minutes between rounds					
287 30-20-10-5 Reps for time of: - row (calories) - alternating dumbbell hang snatch					
288 7 Rounds for time: - 7 handstand push-ups - 7 thrusters - 7 knees-to-elbows - 7 deadlifts - 7 burpees - 7 kettlebell swings - 7 pull-ups					

Work-outs	Day 1 Reps / Time / Weight	Day 2 Reps / Time / Weight	Day 3 Reps / Time / Weight	Day 4 Reps / Time / Weight	Day 5 Reps / Time / Weight
For time: - 15 muscle-ups - 150 double-unders 289 - 12 muscle-ups - 120 double-unders - 9 muscle-ups - 90 double-unders					
For time: - 45 kettlebell swings - 400-m run - 35 kettlebell swings 290 - 800-m run - 25 kettlebell swings - 1,200-m run - 15 kettlebell swings					
For time: - 50 dumbbell snatches - 5 rope climbs, lying to standing - 40 dumbbell snatches - 4 rope climbs, 291 lying to standing - 30 dumbbell snatches - 3 rope climbs, lying to standing - 20 dumbbell snatches - 2 rope climb, lying to standing					

Work-outs	Day 1 Reps / Time / Weight	Day 2 Reps / Time / Weight	Day 3 Reps / Time / Weight	Day 4 Reps / Time / Weight	Day 5 Reps / Time / Weight
292	For time: run 800 meters (or 5 minutes) then, 5 rounds of: 10 push-ups 15 med-ball cleans 15 burpees then, run the same distance					
293	3 Rounds for time of: - run 800 meters - 50 back extensions - 50 sit-ups					
294	3 Rounds for reps in 17 minutes: - 1:00 thrusters - 1:00 power cleans - 1:00 box jump-overs - 1:00 pull-ups - 1:00 assault bike cals - 1:00 rest					
295	Complete as many rounds as possible in 20 minutes of: - 5 pull-ups - 10 push-ups - 15 air squats					

Work-outs	Day 1 Reps / Time / Weight	Day 2 Reps / Time / Weight	Day 3 Reps / Time / Weight	Day 4 Reps / Time / Weight	Day 5 Reps / Time / Weight
For time: - 30 alternating dumbbell snatches - 30 air squats - 30 deadlifts - 30 push-ups - 30 hang cleans - 30 wall ball shots 296 - 30 russian kettlebell swings - 30 box jump overs - 30 shoulder-to-overheads - 30 ball slams - 18 burpees cash-out: 500 meter row					
4 Rounds for time of: 297 - run 400 meters - 30 box step-ups - 30 squats					
Complete as many rounds as possible in 20 minutes of: 298 - 2 muscle-ups - 4 handstand push-ups - 8 kettlebell swings					

Work-outs	Day 1 Reps / Time / Weight	Day 2 Reps / Time / Weight	Day 3 Reps / Time / Weight	Day 4 Reps / Time / Weight	Day 5 Reps / Time / Weight
13 Rounds for time, starting with 1 and adding an exercise each round of: - 1 wall walk - 2 candlesticks - 3 burpees - 4 push-ups - 5 walking lunges - 6 air squats - 7 sit-ups - 8 jumping squats - 9 jumping lunges - 10 broad jumps - 11 handstand push-ups - 12 pistols					
3 Rounds for time: - 25 foot dumbbell overhead walking lunges - 15 calorie assault bike - 25 foot dumbbell overhead walking lunges - 8 toes-to-bars					
Complete as many rounds as possible in 20 minutes of: - 5 pull-ups - 10 push-ups - 15 squats					

Work-outs	Day 1 Reps / Time / Weight	Day 2 Reps / Time / Weight	Day 3 Reps / Time / Weight	Day 4 Reps / Time / Weight	Day 5 Reps / Time / Weight
302 As many reps as possible in 25 minutes: - 5 devil presses - 20 double dumbbell front rack reverse lunges - 25 calorie row					
303 12 Rounds for time: - 12 burpees - 12 air squats - 12 push-ups - 12 sit-ups time cap: 25 minutes					
304 Complete as many rounds as possible in 20 minutes: - 15 sit-ups - 25 burpees - 35 wall-ball shots					
305 5 Rounds for time of: - 10 deadlifts - 10 burpees					

Work-outs	Day 1 Reps / Time / Weight	Day 2 Reps / Time / Weight	Day 3 Reps / Time / Weight	Day 4 Reps / Time / Weight	Day 5 Reps / Time / Weight
Buy-in: 20 burpees every minute on the minute for 20 minutes - minute 1: 15 calorie row - minute 2: 20 plate ground-to-overheads - minute 3: 20 sit-ups - minute 4: 6 devil press thrusters - minute 5: rest repeat x 4					
306 every minute on the minute for 20 minutes - minute 1: 6 kettlebell deadlifts + 6 kettlebell swings + 6 kettlebell thrusters - minute 2: 50 single-unders - minute 3: 12 alternating dumbbell snatches - minute 4: 10 up-downs repeat x 5 buy-out: 18 burpees					
307 For time: 5-10-15-10-5 of - clean - pull-ups					

Work-outs	Day 1 Reps / Time / Weight	Day 2 Reps / Time / Weight	Day 3 Reps / Time / Weight	Day 4 Reps / Time / Weight	Day 5 Reps / Time / Weight
308 Complete as many rounds as possible in 11 minutes of: - 11 dumbbell hang power cleans - 11 assisted push-ups					
309 For time: - 70 sit-ups - 60 toes-to-bars - 50 ghd sit-ups - 40 pull-ups - 30 strict pull-ups - 20 bar muscle-ups					
310 For time: round 1: - 1,000 meter row - 1 mile assault air bike - 200 single-unders round 2: - 750 meter row - 0.5 mile assault air bike - 150 single-unders round 3: - 500 meter row - 0.5 mile assault air bike - 100 single-unders round 4: - 250 meter row - 0.5 mile assault air bike - 50 single-unders					

	Day 1	Day 2	Day 3	Day 4	Day 5
Work-outs	Reps / Time / Weight	Reps / Time / Weight	Reps / Time / Weight	Reps / Time / Weight	Reps / Time / Weight
311 6 Rounds for time: - 6 front squats - 6 pull-ups - 6 bench presses - 6 deadlifts - 6 barbell rows - 6 shoulder-to-overheads					
312 As many reps as possible in 20 minutes: - 25 burpees - 200 meter run - 25 kettlebell swings - 200 meter run - 25 pull-ups - 200 meter run - 25 push-ups - 200 meter run					
313 Every 3 minutes (for 6 rounds) in 20 minutes: - 6 burpees - 18 alternating dumbbell snatches - 8 toes-to-bars - 10 goblet squats					
314 As many reps as possible in 24 minutes: - 6 handstand push-ups - 12 pull-ups - 24 air squats					

Work-outs	Day 1 Reps / Time / Weight	Day 2 Reps / Time / Weight	Day 3 Reps / Time / Weight	Day 4 Reps / Time / Weight	Day 5 Reps / Time / Weight
315	30 Muscle-ups for time if you cannot do the muscle-ups, do 120 pull-ups and 120 dips					
316	As many reps as possible in 15 minutes: - 20 wall ball shots - 20 calorie row					
317	21-15-9 Reps for time: - burpees - kettlebell swings - double-unders					
318	For time: - 20 thrusters - run 200 meters - 25 thrusters - run 400 meters - 30 air squats - run 800 meters					
319	As many reps as possible in 25 minutes: - 5 renegade rows - 10 burpee box jump over - 15 abmat sit ups - 20 dual db overhead walking lunges - 25 double-unders					
320	6 Rounds for time: - 60 double-unders - 30 kettlebell swings - 15 burpees					

	Day 1	Day 2	Day 3	Day 4	Day 5
Work-outs	Reps / Time / Weight	Reps / Time / Weight	Reps / Time / Weight	Reps / Time / Weight	Reps / Time / Weight
321 Complete as many reps as possible in 5 minutes of: - shoulder presses each time you break, perform 50 single-unders rest 3 minutes then, complete as many reps as possible in 5 minutes of: - hang power cleans each time you break, perform 20 squats					
322 For time: - 100 wall-ball shots					
323 As many reps as possible in 18 minutes: - 8 toes-to-bars - 18 overhead squats - 8 floor presses - 18 calorie bike + barbell hold - 36 double-unders					
324 As many reps as possible in 21 minutes: - 7 burpees - 11 push-ups - 22 kettlebell swings buy-in: 65 sit-ups					

Work-outs	Day 1 Reps / Time / Weight	Day 2 Reps / Time / Weight	Day 3 Reps / Time / Weight	Day 4 Reps / Time / Weight	Day 5 Reps / Time / Weight
325 5 Rounds of: - 1 minute of burpees - 1 minute of sit-ups rest 1 minute					
326 As many reps as possible in 20 minutes: - 2 muscle-ups - 4 handstand push-ups - 8 kettlebell swings					
327 Run for 35 minutes. - every 5 minutes, stop and perform 15 burpees.					
328 For time: - 50 air squats - 50 jumping jacks - 50 push-ups - 50 jumping jacks - 50 lunges - 50 jumping jacks - 50 burpees - 50 jumping jacks - 50 mountain climbers (l+r=1) - 50 jumping jacks - 50 mountain climbers (l+r=1) - 50 jumping jacks - 50 burpees - 50 jumping jacks - 50 lunges - 50 jumping jacks - 50 push-ups - 50 jumping jacks - 50 air squats					

Work-outs	Day 1 Reps / Time / Weight	Day 2 Reps / Time / Weight	Day 3 Reps / Time / Weight	Day 4 Reps / Time / Weight	Day 5 Reps / Time / Weight
329 As many repetitions as possible in 5 rounds of: - max bench press (bodyweight) - max pull-ups					
330 For time: 3-9-15-21-15-9-3 - deadlifts - box jumps					
331 For time: - 75 wall-ball shots - 75-cal. row					
332 For time: 50-40-30-20-10 reps of: - calorie row - burpees - alternating lunges					
333 4 Rounds for time of: - 2 rope climbs - 10 dips - 12 abmat sit-ups					
334 For 20 minutes: - 10 dumbbell thrusters - 10 pull-ups					
335 6 Rounds for time: - 35 kettlebell swings - 30 push-ups - 25 pull-ups - 20 box jumps - 1 mile run					
336 15-12-9-6-3 Reps for time of: - power cleans - bar-facing burpees					

Work-outs	Day 1 Reps / Time / Weight	Day 2 Reps / Time / Weight	Day 3 Reps / Time / Weight	Day 4 Reps / Time / Weight	Day 5 Reps / Time / Weight
337 As many reps as possible in 18 minutes: - 300 meter run - 9 deadlift - 6 burpee bar muscle-ups					
338 8 Rounds for time: - 24 air squats - 24 push-ups - 24 walking lunges - 400 meter run					
339 As many reps as possible in 10 minutes: - 5 shoulder-to-overheads - 10 deadlifts - 15 box jumps					
340 As many reps as possible in 10 minutes: - 30 double-unders - 15 power snatches					
341 5 Rounds for time: - 15 deadlifts - 12 hang power cleans - 9 push jerks					
342 Complete as many rounds as possible in 7 minutes of: - 50 double-unders - 10 overhead squats					

Work-outs	Day 1 Reps / Time / Weight	Day 2 Reps / Time / Weight	Day 3 Reps / Time / Weight	Day 4 Reps / Time / Weight	Day 5 Reps / Time / Weight
For time: - 24 back squats - 8 rope climbs - 15 back squats - 5 rope climbs - 12 back squats - 4 rope climbs					
As many reps as possible in 20 minutes: - 10 push presses - 10 kettlebell swings - 10 box jumps					
As many reps as possible in 25 minutes: - 10 pull-ups - 20 push-ups - 30 air squats - 15 pull-ups - 30 push-ups - 45 air squats - 20 pull-ups - 40 push-ups - 60 air squats - 25 pull-ups - 50 push-ups - 75 air squats - 30 pull-ups - 60 push-ups - 90 air squats					

343
344
345

Work-outs	Day 1 Reps / Time / Weight	Day 2 Reps / Time / Weight	Day 3 Reps / Time / Weight	Day 4 Reps / Time / Weight	Day 5 Reps / Time / Weight
346	As many reps as possible in 15 minutes: - 15 air squats - 10 sit-ups - 5 walkouts to push-ups every 2 minutes, complete: - 3 burpees					
347	Complete as many rounds as possible in 15 minutes of: - 5 pull-ups - 10 push-ups - 15 med-ball cleans					
348	3 Rounds for time of: - 15 hand power clean - 15 burpees					
349	As many reps as possible in 21 minutes: - 3 overhead squats - 6 overhead lunges - 9 power snatches - 12 push-ups - 15 calorie assault air bike					

Work-outs	Day 1 Reps / Time / Weight	Day 2 Reps / Time / Weight	Day 3 Reps / Time / Weight	Day 4 Reps / Time / Weight	Day 5 Reps / Time / Weight
Four parts in 12 minutes every minute on the minute for 3 minutes: - 15 dumbbell rows - 10 push-ups every minute on the minute for 3 minutes: 350 - 10 dumbbell rows - 10 push-ups every minute on the minute for 3 minutes: - 15 dumbbell rows - 10 push-ups then, as many reps as possible in 3 minutes: - dumbbell rows					
Four 3-minute rounds - as many reps as possibles in 3 minutes per round: 351 - 7 dumbbell hang power cleans - 7 pull-ups - 7 box jump overs rest 1 minute after each round					
As many reps as possible in 12 minutes: 352 - 7 power cleans - 21 sit-ups - 11 pull-ups - 21 wall ball shots					

Work-outs	Day 1 Reps / Time / Weight	Day 2 Reps / Time / Weight	Day 3 Reps / Time / Weight	Day 4 Reps / Time / Weight	Day 5 Reps / Time / Weight
353 Complete as many rounds as possible in 15 minutes of: - 12 burpees - 12 back squats					
354 3-minute inverted hold of: - 50 squats - 30-meter bear crawl - 50 squats - 30 knee push-ups					
355 Complete as many rounds as possible in 12 minutes of: - 3 ring rows - 6 push-ups - 9 squats					
356 As many reps as possible in 11 minutes: - 1 rope climb - 5 squat snatches - 2 rope climbs - 5 squat snatches continue with this pattern, adding 1 rope climb every round					
357 21-15-9 Reps for time of: - snatches - chest-to-bar pull-ups					
358 As many reps as possible in 15 minutes: - 30 double-unders - 15 power snatches					

	Day 1	Day 2	Day 3	Day 4	Day 5
Work-outs	Reps / Time / Weight	Reps / Time / Weight	Reps / Time / Weight	Reps / Time / Weight	Reps / Time / Weight
359 As many reps as possible in 12 minutes: - 9 thrusters - 21 burpees - 15 kettlebell swings - 1000 meter row					
360 For time: - 20 pull-ups - 50 deadlifts - 50 push-ups - 50 box jumps - 50 floor wipers (one count) - 50 kettlebell clean-and-presses - 20 pull-ups					
361 21-18-15-12-9-6-3 Reps for time of: - front squats - ghd sit-ups					
362 For time: - 10 bench presses - 10 power cleans - 100 meter run - 8 bench presses - 8 power cleans - 100 meter run - 6 bench presses - 6 power cleans - 100 meter run - 4 bench presses - 4 power cleans - 100 meter run - 2 bench presses - 2 power cleans - 100 meter run					

Work-outs	Day 1 Reps / Time / Weight	Day 2 Reps / Time / Weight	Day 3 Reps / Time / Weight	Day 4 Reps / Time / Weight	Day 5 Reps / Time / Weight
As many reps as possible in 13 minutes: 363 - 12 box jumps - 6 thrusters - 6 bar facing burpees					
Three 3-minute rounds of: - 100-m farmers carry 364 then as many reps as possible of: - 3 burpees - 7 kettlebell swings rest 2 minutes between rounds					
4 Rounds for time of: 365 - 400 meter run - 1-minute plank hold					
As many reps as possible in 15 minutes: 366 - 5 muscle-ups - 50 wall ball shots - 100 double-unders					

Work-outs	Day 1 Reps / Time / Weight	Day 2 Reps / Time / Weight	Day 3 Reps / Time / Weight	Day 4 Reps / Time / Weight	Day 5 Reps / Time / Weight
367 As many reps as possible in 15 minutes: 3 rounds of: - 10 toes-to-bars - 15 sumo deadlift high-pulls - 15 push presses - 10 bar-over burpees then, in remaining time: - max calorie assault air bike					
368 20 Rounds for time: - 15 kettlebell swings - 5 goblet squats - 3 push-ups					
369 For time: - 20 jumping bar muscle-ups - 5 overhead squats - 10 jumping bar muscle-ups - 10 overhead squats - 5 jumping bar muscle-ups - 20 overhead squats					
370 As many reps as possible in 22 minutes: - 22 wall ball shots - 22 power snatches - 22 box jumps - 22 push presses - 22 calorie row					

Work-outs	Day 1 Reps / Time / Weight	Day 2 Reps / Time / Weight	Day 3 Reps / Time / Weight	Day 4 Reps / Time / Weight	Day 5 Reps / Time / Weight
8 Rounds for time: - 8 push-ups - 8 ghd sit-ups - 8 air squats - 8 pull-ups 371 - 8 deadlifts - 8 hang power cleans - 8 shoulder-to-overheads - 8 calorie row					
21-15-9 Reps for time: 372 - thrusters - pull-ups					
As many reps as possible in 25 minutes: 373 - 5 pull-ups - 10 push-ups - 15 squats - 5 pull-ups - 10 thrusters					
For time: - 5 sets of: 4 pull-ups + 4 push-ups 374 - 50 squats - 5 sets of: 4 pull-ups + 4 push-ups - 50-calorie row					
For time: - 1-3-6-9-15-21 wall walks 375 - 10-30-60-90-150-210 double-unders time cap: 16 minutes					

Work-outs	Day 1 Reps / Time / Weight	Day 2 Reps / Time / Weight	Day 3 Reps / Time / Weight	Day 4 Reps / Time / Weight	Day 5 Reps / Time / Weight
376 As many reps as possible in 20 minutes: - 20 calorie assault air bike - 20 kettlebell swings - 20 abmat sit-ups					
377 7 Rounds for time of: - 15 ghd sit-ups - 15 back extensions - 10 thrusters - 10 clean and jerks					
378 5 Rounds for time of: - 100-ft. handstand walk - 30 single-leg squats, alternating					
379 6 Rounds for time: - 30 double-unders - 20 knees-to-elbows - 10 handstand push-ups					
380 50 Rounds for time: - 1 burpee - 1 push-up - 1 jumping-jack - 1 sit-up - 1 handstand					
381 4 Rounds for time of: - 12-calorie row - 9 hang power snatches - 6 burpees					

	Day 1	Day 2	Day 3	Day 4	Day 5
Work-outs	Reps / Time / Weight	Reps / Time / Weight	Reps / Time / Weight	Reps / Time / Weight	Reps / Time / Weight
382 With a running clock in 15 minutes: from 0:00-3:00, complete: - 500 meter row in the remaining time, as many reps as possible of: - 9 dumbbell thrusters - 18 chest-to-bar pull-ups - 9 devil presses					
383 6 Rounds for time: - 6 power cleans - 12 front squats - 6 jerks - 24 pull-ups 90 seconds rest					
384 As many reps as possible in 10 minutes: - 10 power cleans - 10 burpees over the bar - 20 deadlifts - 20 pull-ups					
385 For time: - 500 meter row - 40 air squats - 30 sit-ups - 20 push-ups - 10 pull-ups					

	Day 1	Day 2	Day 3	Day 4	Day 5
Work-outs	Reps / Time / Weight	Reps / Time / Weight	Reps / Time / Weight	Reps / Time / Weight	Reps / Time / Weight
386 For time: buy-in: - 250 meter run then, 5 rounds of: - 10 lunges - 10 air squats - 10 sit-ups - 10 burpees cash-out: - 250 meter run					
387 10 Rounds for time: - 25 foot handstand walk - 5 snatches - 7 ring muscle-ups - 25 foot handstand walk					
388 As many reps as possible in 8 minutes: - 3 clean-and-jerks - 3 toes-to-bars - 6 clean-and-jerks - 6 toes-to-bars - 9 clean-and-jerks - 9 toes-to-bars - 12 clean-and-jerks - 12 toes-to-bars					
389 20 Minute as many reps as possible: - 14 v-ups - 7 burpees - 14 plank shoulder taps - 7 burpees - 14 windshield wipers - 7 burpees					

Work-outs	Day 1 Reps / Time / Weight	Day 2 Reps / Time / Weight	Day 3 Reps / Time / Weight	Day 4 Reps / Time / Weight	Day 5 Reps / Time / Weight
390 For time: - 100 deadlifts - 100 power cleans - 100 ground-to-overheads - 50 burpees					
391 As many reps as possible in 22 minutes: - 200 meter run - 100 double-unders - 30 burpees - 4 rope climbs					
392 For time: 20-16-12-8-4 reps of: - bench presses - calorie row					
393 As many reps as possible 15 minutes: - 6 deadlifts - 9 bar-facing burpees - 9 bar muscle-ups					
394 Complete as many reps as possible in 15 minutes of: - run 200 meters - 15 ring rows					
395 For time: - 10 thrusters - 15 bar-facing burpees - 20 thrusters - 25 bar-facing burpees - 30 thrusters - 35 bar-facing burpees					

Work-outs	Day 1 Reps / Time / Weight	Day 2 Reps / Time / Weight	Day 3 Reps / Time / Weight	Day 4 Reps / Time / Weight	Day 5 Reps / Time / Weight
396	3 Rounds for total reps in 18 minutes: - 1 minute burpees - 1 minute power snatches - 1 minute box jumps - 1 minute thrusters - 1 minute chest-to-bar pull-ups - 1 minute rest					
397	5 Rounds of: - 5 burpees - 20 squats - 5 burpees - 10 push ups - 5 burpees - 20 lunges - 5 burpees - 10 v-ups					
398	For time: - 50 burpees - 500 meter run - 100 push-ups - 500 meter run - 150 walking lunges - 500 meter run - 200 air squats - 500 meter run - 150 walking lunges - 500 meter run - 100 push-ups - 500 meter run - 50 burpees					

Work-outs	Day 1 Reps / Time / Weight	Day 2 Reps / Time / Weight	Day 3 Reps / Time / Weight	Day 4 Reps / Time / Weight	Day 5 Reps / Time / Weight
399 10 Rounds for time: - 3 devil presses - 22 alternating dumbbell lunges - 19 air squats					
400 As many reps as possible in 7 minutes: - burpees					
401 As many reps as possible in 35 minutes: buy-in: - 9 man makers - 11 burpees in remaining time, as many reps as possible of: - 300 meter run - 30 air squats - 10 handstand push-ups					
402 7 Rounds for time: - 10 push-ups - 10 air squats - run 200m					
403 Complete as many rounds as possible in 12 minutes of: - 3 burpee box jump-overs - 3 deadlifts - 6 burpee box jump-overs - 6 deadlifts - 9 burpee box jump-overs - 9 deadlifts etc.					

	Day 1 Reps / Time / Weight	Day 2 Reps / Time / Weight	Day 3 Reps / Time / Weight	Day 4 Reps / Time / Weight	Day 5 Reps / Time / Weight
Work-outs					
404 4 Rounds for time: - 1 deadlift - 2 muscle-ups - 3 squat cleans - 4 handstand push ups					
405 4 Rounds for time: - 14 push-ups - 14 sit-ups - 14 box jumps - 14 kettlebell swings - 14 push presses - 14 walking lunges (each leg) - 14 mountain climbers - 14 knees-to-elbows - 14 pull-ups - 14 parallel bar dips - 14 air squats - 14 back extensions - 14 burpees					
406 10 Rounds for time of: - 100-m sprint - 5 burpees - 20 sit-ups - 15 push-ups - 100-m sprint rest 2 minutes					

Work-outs	Day 1 Reps / Time / Weight	Day 2 Reps / Time / Weight	Day 3 Reps / Time / Weight	Day 4 Reps / Time / Weight	Day 5 Reps / Time / Weight
407 As many reps as possible in 23 minutes: - 23 air squats - 23 push-ups - 23 kettlebell swings - 23 jumping lunges - 23 sit-ups - 23 box jumps					
408 For time: - 25 toes-to-bars - 50-calorie row - 75 push-ups - 50 box jumps - 25 pull-ups					
409 10 Rounds for time: - 4 snatches - 4 bar over burpees					
410 Four 3-minute rounds of: - 100-meter dumbbell farmers carry then as many reps as possible of: - 10 push-ups - 10 dumbbell squats rest 1 minutes between rounds					

Work-outs	Day 1 Reps / Time / Weight	Day 2 Reps / Time / Weight	Day 3 Reps / Time / Weight	Day 4 Reps / Time / Weight	Day 5 Reps / Time / Weight
411 Five 3-minute as many reps as possibles in 19 minutes as many reps as possible in 3 minutes - 3 power cleans - 6 push-ups - 9 air squats then rest 1 minute repeat 5 times					
412 As many rounds as possible in 21 minutes: - 30 calorie row - 20 burpees over rower - 10 power cleans					
413 5 Rounds for time: - 600 meter run - 30 kettlebell swings - 30 pull-ups					
414 For time: - row 1,000 meters - 50 dumbbell squat snatches, alternating - row 750 meters - 35 dumbbell squat snatches, alternating - row 500 meters - 20 dumbbell squat snatches, alternating					

Work-outs	Day 1 Reps / Time / Weight	Day 2 Reps / Time / Weight	Day 3 Reps / Time / Weight	Day 4 Reps / Time / Weight	Day 5 Reps / Time / Weight
415 3 Rounds for time of: - 30 sit-ups - 500-meter run					
416 30-20-10 Reps for time of: - toes-to-bars - kettlebell walking lunges					
417 For time: - 30 snatches					
418 2 Rounds for time: - 25 deadlifts - 25 box jumps - 25 wall ball shots - 25 bench press - 25 box jumps - 25 wall ball shots - 25 cleans					
419 As many reps as possible in 30 minutes: - 30 air squats - 20 box jumps - 30 meter walking lunges - 20 hand release push-ups - 30 burpees - 100 meter run					
420 As many reps as possible in 20 minutes: - 5 pull-ups - 10 push-ups - 15 air squats - 20 calorie row					

Work-outs	Day 1 Reps / Time / Weight	Day 2 Reps / Time / Weight	Day 3 Reps / Time / Weight	Day 4 Reps / Time / Weight	Day 5 Reps / Time / Weight
421 For time: - 20 hanging knee raises - 20 single-arm dumbbell snatches - 20 dumbbell box step-overs - 20 single-arm dumbbell snatches - 20 hanging knee raises					
422 4 Rounds For Time: - 2 jerks - 10 toes-to-bars - 2 jerks - 10 kettlebell swings					
423 For time: - 1 mile run - 2,000 meter row - 1 mile run					
424 4 Rounds for time of: - run 400 meters - 30 back squats					
425 As many reps as possible in 15 minutes: - 5 handstand push-ups - 10 pull-ups - 15 push-ups					
426 9-6-3 Reps for time of: - snatch - burpee box step-over					

Work-outs	Day 1 Reps / Time / Weight	Day 2 Reps / Time / Weight	Day 3 Reps / Time / Weight	Day 4 Reps / Time / Weight	Day 5 Reps / Time / Weight
As many reps as possible in 10 minutes: - 30 snatches - 30 snatches (increased weight) - 30 snatches ((increased weight)					
4 Rounds for time: - 400 meter run - 16 bench presses - 16 wall ball shots - 16 shoulder-to-overheads - 16 ghd sit-ups					
10 Rounds for time: - 10 thrusters - 35 double-unders time cap: 40 minutes					
For time: - 2 minute elbow plank - 13 burpees - 18 kettlebell swings - 31 push-ups - 53 goblet squats - 53 burpees - 31 kettlebell swings - 18 push-ups - 13 goblet squats - 2 minute wall sit					

427
428
429
430

	Day 1	Day 2	Day 3	Day 4	Day 5
Work-outs	Reps / Time / Weight	Reps / Time / Weight	Reps / Time / Weight	Reps / Time / Weight	Reps / Time / Weight
431 As many reps as possible in 22 minutes: - 22 dumbbell snatches - 4 man makers - 22 burpees - 22 single dumbbell front squats					
432 For time: - 1,000 box step-ups - wear a ruck pack					
433 Complete as many rounds in 12 minutes as you can of: - 6 front squats - 12 chest-to-bar pull-ups - 24 double-unders					
434 3 Rounds for time: - 12 deadlifts - 9 hang power cleans - 6 bar facing burpees					
435 4 Rounds for time of: - 20 power snatches - 50 double-unders					
436 3 Rounds for time: - 50 air squats - 5 muscle-ups - 10 hang power cleans					

Work-outs	Day 1 Reps / Time / Weight	Day 2 Reps / Time / Weight	Day 3 Reps / Time / Weight	Day 4 Reps / Time / Weight	Day 5 Reps / Time / Weight
437 4 Rounds for time: - 20 kettlebell ground-to-overheads - 20 kettlebell front squats - 20 kettlebell push-ups (each hand) - 400 meter kettlebell run					
438 6 Rounds for time of: - 30 squats - 20 power cleans - 10 strict pull-ups - run 500 meters					
439 8 Rounds for time: - 400 meter run - 30 back squats					
440 For time: - 60 hip-back extensions each time you break a set or rest at the bottom, stop and perform 15 wall-ball shots. rest 60 seconds after each set of wall-ball shots.					

Work-outs	Day 1 Reps / Time / Weight	Day 2 Reps / Time / Weight	Day 3 Reps / Time / Weight	Day 4 Reps / Time / Weight	Day 5 Reps / Time / Weight
441 As many reps as possible in 20 minutes: - 25 burpees - 200 meter run - 25 kettlebell swings - 200 meter run - 25 pull-ups - 200 meter run - 25 push-ups - 200 meter run					
442 3 Rounds for time of: - run 800 meters - 50 sit-ups					
443 Complete as many rounds as possible in 8 minutes of: - 10 back squats - 10 strict chest-to-bar pull-ups					
444 5-4-3-2-1 Reps for time of: - 15-ft. rope climbs - clean and jerks					
445 4 Rounds for time of: - run 200 meters - 20 squats - 15 push presses					
446 3 Rounds for time of: - 500-m row - 25 thrusters - 15 pull-ups					

Work-outs	Day 1 Reps / Time / Weight	Day 2 Reps / Time / Weight	Day 3 Reps / Time / Weight	Day 4 Reps / Time / Weight	Day 5 Reps / Time / Weight
As many reps as possible in 11 minutes: 447 - 11 overhead squats - 11 ball slams - 11 wall ball shots - 11 russian kettlebell swings					
As many reps as possible in 25 minutes: 448 - 10 pull-ups - 15 kettlebell swings - 20 box jumps					
Complete as many rounds as possible in 12 minutes of: 449 - 3 snatches - 6 clean and jerks - 9 ring rows - 60 single-unders					
For time: - 60 hang power snatches 450 - 50 push presses - 40 sumo deadlift high pulls - 30 front squats					

BONUS No 2 - VIDEOS for ALL EXERCISES ARE AVAILABLE if you want check how the exercises are to be performed. The QR codes are shown on the following pages

Abmat sit ups

Air squats

Alternating dumbbell hang snatch

Alternating dumbbell lunges

Alternating dumbbell snatches

Alternating jumping lunges

Alternating kettlebell clean and presses

Alternating lunges

Alternating Split
Squat Jumps

Assault Bike

Back Extensions

Back Squat

Ball Slams

Bar Facing
Burpees

Bar Hang

Bar Muscle Ups

Bar Over Burpees

Barbell Rows

Bear Crawl

Bench Presses

Bent Over Rows

Bicep Curls

Box Jump

Box Jump Overs

Box Step Ups

Broad Jump

Burpee Box Jump Overs

Burpee Box Jumps

Burpee Box Step Over

Burpee Muscle Ups

Burpee Pull Ups

Burpees

Burpees Over The Bar

Calorie Assault Air Bike

Calorie Row

Calorie Ski

Candlesticks

Chest To Bar Pull-Ups

Clean and Jerks

Cleans

Crunches

Curtis p

Deadlift

Deficit Handstand
Push-Ups

Devil Press
Thrusters

Devil Presses

Double Dumbbell
Front Rack Reverse
Lunges

Double Kettlebell
Swings

Double Under

Downward Dog Foot Taps

Dual Dumbbell Overhead Walking Lunges

Dumbbell Box Step Overs

Dumbbell Deadlifts

Dumbbell Farmers Carry

Dumbbell Floor Presses

Dumbbell Front Squats

Dumbbell Front Rack Lunge

Dumbbell Hang Clean Thrusters

Dumbbell Hang Power Cleans

Dumbbell Man Makers

Dumbbell Overhead Lunge

Dumbbell Overhead Walking Lunges

Dumbbell Power Cleans

Dumbbell Push Jerks

Dumbbell Push Presses

Dumbbell Rows

Dumbbell Snatches

Dumbbell Squat Cleans

Dumbbell Squats

Dumbbell Sumo Cleans

Dumbbell Thrusters

Dumbbell Walking Lunges

Elbow Plank

Elbow Plank To Push-Ups

Elevated Push-Ups

Farmer Carry

Fat Bar Thrusters

Floor Wipers

Front Squats

GHD Sit-Ups

Goblet Squats

Ground to Overheads

Hand Release Push-Ups

Handstand

Handstand Push-Ups

Handstand Walk

Hang Cleans

Hang Power Cleans

Hang Power Snatches

Hang Snatches

Hang Squat Cleans

Hanging Knee Raises

High Knees

Hip Extensions

Hip-back Extensions

Hollow Hold

Hollow Rocks

Jerks

Jumping Bar
Muscle-Ups

Jumping Chest To
Bar Pull-Ups

Jumping Jacks

Jumping Lunges

Jumping Pull-Ups

Jumping Squats

Kettlebell Clean And Presses

Kettlebell Deadlifts

Kettlebell Front Squats

Kettlebell Goblet Squats

Kettlebell Ground To Overheads

Kettlebell Push-Ups

Kettlebell Snatches

Kettlebell Sumo Deadlift High-Pulls

Kettlebell Swings

Kettlebell Taters

Kettlebell Thrusters

Kettlebell Walking Lunges

Knee Push-Ups

Knee Raises

Knees To Elbows

Left-Hand Turkish Get-Ups

L-Sit

Lunge

Man Makers

Medball Ball Facing Burpees

Med Ball Cleans

Med Ball Overhead Walking Lunges

Medicine Ball Sit-Ups

Medicine Ball Cleans

Mountain Climbers

Muscle-Ups

Overhead Squats

Overhead Walking Lunge

Overhead Walking Lunges

Parallel Bar Dips

Pendlay Rows

Pistols

Plank Hold

Plank Shoulder Taps

Plate Ground To
Overheads

Plate Overhead
Lunges

Power Cleans

Power Snatches

Pull-Ups

Push Jerks

Push Presses

Push-Ups

Renegade Rows

Right-Hand Turkish
Get-Ups

Ring Dips

Ring Rows

Rope Climbs

Row

Russian Kettlebell
Swings

Seated Leg Raises

Second Hollow Hold

Shoulder Press

Shoulder Taps

Shoulder To
Overhead

Shuttle Runs

Single Dumbbell
Front Squats

Single-Arm Dumbbell Overhead Walking Lunges

Single-Arm Dumbbell Snatches

Single-Arm Dumbbell Thrusters

Single-Arm Overhead Walking Lunges

Single-Leg Squat

Single-Unders

Sit-Ups

Ski Erg

Skull Crushers

Snatches

Squat Cleans

Squat Jumps

Squat Snatches

Squats

Step-Ups

Straight Leg Sit-Ups

Strict Chest-To Bar
Pull-Ups

Strict Pull-Ups

Strict Ring Dips

Sumo Deadlift High
Pulls

Thrusters

Toes-To-Bars

Tp-Downs

Tuck Jumps

Tuck Ups

V-Ups

Waiter Walk

Walking Lunge,
Weight Back-Racked

Walking Lunge,
Weight Front-Racked

Walking Lunge,
Weight Overhead

Walking Lunge

Walking Lunge Steps

Walking Lunges	Walkouts To Push-Ups

Wall Ball Shots	Wall Walk

Weighted Run	Windshield Wipers